Protect yourself from dementia

12 easy natural steps, based on clinical studies, to lower your risk for dementia and Alzheimer's

Graham Fysh

LifeTime Creations

WHY YOU SHOULD CARE

Dementia Is A Major Health Care Issue

Dementia is a major cause of dependency and disability among older people around the world.

Nearly half of all older adults now die with a diagnosis of dementia listed on their medical record, according to a study at the University of Michigan Medicine.

Already dementia is the seventh biggest killer globally. It seems to be becoming worse. The number of people worldwide who will be diagnosed with dementia is expected to double from 57.4 million in 2019 to 152.8 million in 2050.

Dementia is the biggest health and social care issue of our time, says James White, who heads the Alzheimer Society's National Influencing department. Alzheimer's is the most common form of dementia, accounting for 60 percent to 80 percent of dementia cases.

The individual and economic devastation caused by dementia shows no sign of stopping, adds White.

The Alzheimer's Association says that more than 6.5 million Americans are living with Alzheimer's disease and one in three seniors die with the disease or another form of dementia.

Increasing Once More

A study in the United States found that the number of dementia cases among people older than 65 fell from 2000 to 2016. But the number of cases is growing again globally. So much so that scientists now predict a future in which there will be significantly more dementia cases than now.

A new study by the University College London estimates that 1.7 million people could be dealing with the condition in Britain by 2040. Overall, the number of dementia cases could be 42 percent higher than previous studies had predicted, the study says.

"It is shocking to think that the number of people living with dementia by 2040 might be up to 70 percent higher than if dementia cases had continued to decline," says Dr. Yuntao Chen, who was lead author of the study.

"Not only will this have a devastating effect on the lives of those involved but it will also put a considerably larger burden on health and social care than current forecasts predict," Chen says.

Dementia is likely to be a more urgent policy problem than recognized until now, says Professor Eric Brunner who was principal investigator of the study.

Not only that, but people with dementia, who are the biggest users of social care, are struggling with a health care system that is costly, difficult to access, and too often not tailored to their needs, White of the Alzheimer Society says.

Greater Attention On Prevention

A cure for dementia and Alzheimer's remains elusive, however. So far, medications that have been developed have been largely unsuccessful.

Without a cure on the horizon, medical researchers are now placing greater attention on prevention as the best way to tackle this disabling condition.

As a result, medical research is aimed at promoting healthy brain aging—and therefore lowering the risk of dementia—through various strategies.

The latest clinical research suggests that you should take steps *before* you face the risk of contracting dementia. In that way you can reduce your risk of contracting the condition later in life.

Although the earlier you start the better, research shows that you can take these steps even when you are becoming older. In some cases clinical studies indicate that taking them when you have early signs of dementia might help to delay the condition and prevent it from becoming worse.

In this report we look at recent scientific findings from around the world that you might find useful if you are seeking to lower your risk of dementia as you age. The best part of these findings is that most of them concern natural steps that you can take. No drugs are involved. Following the advice is likely also to improve your overall health.

STEP ONE

Eat Foods Rich In Magnesium

Adding more magnesium to your daily diet can help you to reduce your risk of dementia, according to scientists at the Neuroimaging and Brain Lab at the Australian National University (ANU).

They suggest that you should obtain this increased magnesium through eating more foods that are rich in magnesium rather than through taking pills.

"Our study shows a 41 per cent increase in magnesium intake could lead to less age-related brain shrinkage, which is associated with better cognitive function and lower the risk or delayed onset of dementia in later life," says the study's lead author Dr. Khawlah Alateeq, from the ANU National Centre for Epidemiology and Population Health.

The research highlights the benefits of a diet that is high in magnesium and the part it plays in promoting good brain health, she adds.

The study researchers say that if we include more magnesium in our diets when we are younger we are more likely to safeguard against cognitive decline by the time we reach our forties.

"This means people of all ages should be paying closer attention to their magnesium intake," says Alateeq.

Women More Than Men

An interesting aspect of this study is that the researchers found that magnesium seemed to benefit women more than men. The benefit was seen most in post-menopausal women than pre-menopausal, although this might be due to the anti-inflammatory effect of magnesium.

Magnesium is a mineral that is present naturally in many foods. In their study, the researchers say they focused on leafy green vegetables, legumes, nuts, seeds and whole grains to provide an average estimate of magnesium intake from the participants' diets.

Here is a closer look at those foods that are high in magnesium and were referred to in the study:

· Seeds and nuts
Pumpkin seeds are the richest in magnesium, followed by Chia seeds. Also high in magnesium are cashews, almonds, peanuts, and flaxseed.

· Legumes
Black beans are tops, followed by Edamame (soy beans) and lima beans.

· Whole grains
Shredded wheat and quinoa in particular have fairly large amounts of magnesium.

· Leafy greens
Highest in magnesium among the dark and leafy greens is spinach, followed by Swiss chard and collard greens.

· Others
Magnesium also is present in bananas, papayas, avocados and blackberries as well as potatoes, peas, and corn.

Dieticians suggest that you obtain your magnesium only from food. Supplements might be prescribed by doctors in some cases but consuming too much magnesium taken in pill form can cause you to suffer side effects, they explain.

How The Study Was Conducted

Those who took part in the study completed an online questionnaire five times over a period of 16 months.

The researchers used the responses to calculate the daily magnesium intake of the participants. They were based on 200 different foods with varying portions.

The university team focused on magnesium-rich foods such as legumes, nuts, seeds, leafy green vegetables and whole grains to provide an average estimate of the magnesium content that was in the participants' diets.

The study appears in the *European Journal of Nutrition*.

STEP TWO

Boost your levels of vitamin D

A world-first study at the University of South Australia found a direct link between dementia and the lack of vitamin D. The study found:

• Lower levels of vitamin D were linked with lower brain volumes and a greater risk of dementia and stroke;

• Genetic analyses supported a link between vitamin D deficiency and dementia;

• As many as 17 percent of dementia cases might be prevented by boosting your levels of vitamin D to normal levels (50 nmol/L).

"Vitamin D is a hormone precursor that is increasingly recognized for widespread effects, including on brain health, but until now it has been very difficult to examine what would happen if we were able to prevent vitamin D deficiency," says Professor Elina Hyppönen, senior investigator and director of UniSA's Australian Centre for Precision Health.

"Our study is the first to examine the effect of very low levels of vitamin D on the risks of dementia and stroke, using robust genetic analyses among a large population."

'Incredibly Significant'

She adds that the findings are "incredibly significant" in light of the high prevalence of dementia around the world.

"Dementia is a progressive and debilitating disease that can devastate individuals and families alike," Hyppönen says. "If we're able to change this reality through ensuring that none of us is severely vitamin D sufficient it would also have further benefits and we could change the health and wellbeing for thousands.

"Most of us are likely to be OK, but for anyone who for whatever reason may not receive enough vitamin D from the sun, modifications to diet may not be enough, and supplementation may well be needed."

Translation: Take vitamin D pills if your vitamin D levels are low and you are unable to spend time in the sun.

How The Study Was Conducted

The study analyzed data from 294,514 participants in the UK Biobank. The researchers examined the impact of low levels of vitamin D (25 mol/L) and the risk of dementia and stroke.

Nonlinear Mendelian randomization—a way of measuring changes in genes to examine the causal effect of a modifiable exposure on disease—was used to test for underlying causes for the impact on the brain, including dementia and stroke.

The study is published in the *American Journal of Clinical Nutrition*.

STEP THREE

Follow a healthy eating pattern

Two studies have found that keeping to a healthy diet can help a lot in keeping dementia at bay.

In the following pages we outline each of them. You choose which diet you prefer.

1. Switch To The D-A-S-H Diet

The first study finds that if women switch during mid-life to the DASH diet they will improve their brain function later in life. They are less likely to report memory loss and other signs of cognitive decline.

The study was held at the New York University's Grossman School of Medicine. It concentrated on women because they make up more than two-thirds of those diagnosed with Alzheimer's disease.

When people start complaining about their daily brain performance, these are signs of more serious brain disorders, such as Alzheimer's, says Dr. Yu Chen, professor in the Department of Population Health and senior author of the study.

"With more than 30 years follow-up, we found that the stronger the adherence to a DASH diet in midlife, the less likely women are to report cognitive issues much later in life," she adds.

"Our data suggest that it is important to start a healthy diet in mid-life to prevent cognitive impairment in older age," says Yixiao Song, a lead author of the study.

The DASH diet (which stands for Dietary Approaches to Stop

Hypertension) was originally designed for people suffering from high blood pressure. It is, however, increasingly being viewed as a healthy diet for other ailments, too. We can now add dementia to that list. Indeed, Dr. Fen Wu, a senior associate research scientist who co-led this study, confirms that following the DASH diet might not only prevent high-blood pressure, but also cognitive issues.

Not only that, but the researchers in this study say that high blood pressure itself, particularly when suffered in midlife, is a risk factor for cognitive decline and dementia.

The DASH diet includes a significant consumption of plant-based foods that are rich in potassium, calcium and magnesium. It concentrates on fruits, vegetables and whole grains. Included are low-fat dairy products, fat-free products, poultry, fish, nuts and beans. It limits saturated fat, cholesterol, sodium and sugar. The diet restricts foods that are high in salt. It also limits saturated fat —as in full-fat dairy products and fatty meats—and added sugar and saturated fat.

How The Study Was Conducted

The researchers analyzed data from 5,116 of the more than 14,000 women enrolled in the New York University Women's Health Study, one of the longest running studies of its kind that examines the impact of lifestyle and other factors on the most common cancers among women, as well as other chronic conditions.

Those who took part in the study filled in questionnaires between 1985 and 1991 when they enrolled in the study and were, on average, 49. These participants were followed for more than 30 years until they reached an average age of 79. They were then asked to report any cognitive complaints.

These complaints were assessed using six standard questions that indicate mild brain impairment, which leads to dementia. The questions related to difficulties in remembering recent events or shopping lists, understanding spoken instructions or group conversations, or navigating familiar streets.

Those women who kept most closely to the DASH diet showed a 17 percent reduction in the odds of reporting multiple cognitive complaints.

The study appears in *Alzheimer's & Dementia,* the journal of the Alzheimer's Association.

ΔΔΔ

2. Switch To A Mediterranean-Based Ketogenic Diet

The second study under the category of eating healthy food comes from researchers at Wake Forest University School of Medicine in North Carolina. It suggests that you can cut your risk of Alzheimer's by following what the researchers call a modified Mediterranean ketogenic diet.

Let's break that down and see what it means.

Firstly, a ketogenic diet means eating an extremely low number of carbohydrates. At the same time, you eat a lot of fat. The theory is that you burn the fat rather than the carbohydrates for energy.

In the keto diet you also focus a lot on meat, whether it be chicken, pork or steak. It also can include nuts, seafood, vegetables and healthy fats from eggs and cheese.

The keto diet is said to lower blood sugar and insulin levels and shifts the body's metabolism away from carbs and toward fat and ketones. It is also said to be good for weight loss.

A Mediterranean diet is less definitive but it is based on plant food. It is high in fruits, vegetables, whole grains, beans, nuts and seeds. It limits consumption of red meat, but includes fish and poultry. It is considered good for lowering your risk of stroke or heart disease.

The researchers compared a low-fat diet with one that consists of healthy fats and protein and low carbohydrates, which they call the modified Mediterranean ketogenic diet. They found that the modified diet showed significant changes in a biological pathway that is linked to Alzheimer's disease.

"We hope that better understanding of this complex relationship between diet, cognitive status and gut health will lead to new interventions to prevent and treat Alzheimer's disease," says Dr. Suzanne Craft, professor of gerontology and geriatric medicine at Wake Forest University School of Medicine.

The study found generally that the modified ketogenic diet might help to prevent cognitive decline—meaning that it can help to avoid the onset of dementia as well as Alzheimer's disease.

The Mediterranean diet is generally high in: Fruits, vegetables, whole grains, nuts and seeds, beans, olive oil, and seasoning with herbs and spices.

The main steps to take to follow the diet include:

• Eat vegetables, fruits, whole grains and plant-based fats daily.

• Each week eat fish, poultry, beans, legumes and eggs.

• Consume moderate portions of dairy products.

• Limit how much red meat you eat.

• Limit how many foods with added sugar you eat.

How The Study Was Conducted

The research team tested their theory on 20 adults, nine of whom were diagnosed with mild cognitive impairment and 11 with normal cognition. They could choose whether they wanted to follow the low-carb modified Mediterranean-ketogenic diet or a low-fat diet higher in carbohydrates. After six weeks, they switched to the other diet.

Stool samples were gathered from the participants at the beginning and end of each diet period to analyze changes in the gut microbiome—the good and the bad bacteria that live in the gastrointestinal tract.

They found that those on the modified Mediterranean ketogenic diet fared better when it came to stopping cognitive decline and boosting brain health than those on the other low-fat and higher carbs diet.

The study also appears in *Alzheimer's & Dementia,* the journal of the Alzheimer's Association.

STEP FOUR

Avoid Alcohol

Even modest amounts of alcohol can speed up the loss of brain cells, according to another study at the Wake Forest University School of Medicine in North Carolina.

Alcohol also increases the number of amyloid plaques, which are the accumulation of toxic proteins found in Alzheimer's disease, the university researchers say.

"These findings suggest alcohol might accelerate the pathological cascade of Alzheimer's disease in its early stages," says Dr. Shannon Macauley, associate professor of physiology and pharmacology at Wake Forest University School of Medicine.

Macauley noted that the study shows that even moderate drinking of alcohol can result in brain injury. Avoiding alcohol will lower your risk of developing dementia and Alzheimer's disease, she added.

Another finding in the study was that moderate alcohol use caused increased anxiety as well as dementia-related behavior.

How The Study Was Conducted

The researchers conducted their experiments on mice.

The mice were given the choice of drinking water or alcohol. In this way, the research team mimicked human behavior when it comes to drinking alcohol. The researchers then studied the effect that voluntary, moderate drinking had on the early stages of

Alzheimer's disease.

They found that alcohol increased brain decay and the number of amyloid plaques, setting the stage for increased numbers of plaque in later life which have been linked to dementia.

The study appears in the journal *Neurobiology of Disease*.

STEP FIVE

Avoid Processed Foods

This study builds on those relating to eating healthy food. It finds that you can lower your chances of developing dementia by changing from high-processed foods to those that are unprocessed. The study was conducted at Tianjin Medical University in China.

The study shows that even relatively small switches in your diet can lower your risk of developing the condition. Such a change can be eating half an apple for lunch, for example, instead of potato chips.

The researchers explain that ultra-processed foods are high in sugar, fat, and salt. They also are lower in fiber and protein.

Such foods, the study says, are cookies, chips, sugary snacks, soft drinks, sausage, ice cream, yogurt, deep-fried chicken, canned baked beans, mayonnaise, canned tomatoes, packaged hummus, ketchup, flavored cereals, packaged guacamole and packaged breads.

You get the picture.

Designed To Be Convenient

Such food is designed to be convenient and easy, says Dr. Huiping Li of Tianjin Medical University.

In addition to salt, fat, and sugar, ultra-processed food also might contain molecules that derive from the packaging or that are produced during heating, Li adds.

Not only that. They usually also contain food additives, which have been shown in earlier studies to harm your thinking or memory abilities.

If you switch from eating these ultra-processed foods and replace them with healthy food choices you will lower your risk of dementia by 20 percent, the researchers found.

Such healthy choices would include fresh fruit, vegetables, beans, milk and meat.

Even Small Changes Can Help

If you boost your consumption of foods that are minimally processed or unprocessed by only 50 grams a day you can cut your risk of developing dementia by 3 percent, the research found.

An amount of 50 grams is equivalent to a serving of fish sticks or a chocolate bar. The unprocessed replacement would be a serving of half an apple, a serving of corn, or a bowl of bran cereal.

It is encouraging, Li says, that even such small and manageable changes in your diet can cut the risk that a person might contract dementia.

Clearly, by making more significant changes in your diet you can cut your risk even further.

How To Decide?

A problem that arises is that some food that is highly processed is actually good for you. How, then, do you know what is highly processed and bad for you and what is highly processed but good for you?

In an editorial that accompanied the study, Dr. Maura E. Walker of Boston University cites an example of food such as soup. It would be classified differently if the soup were homemade or if it were sold in a store in a can. Also, the degree to which the food is processed is not necessarily the same as the quality of the food.

She also uses the example of plant-based burgers that are rated as being of high quality but are highly processed.

In any event, you probably have a good understanding of what constitutes the difference between the two types of processed foods—good versus bad. And which to avoid.

How The Study Was Conducted

The study used records of 18,021 people in Britain's Biobank which is a large database stretching back years containing information on the health of people in the United Kingdom.

Those who were studied were older than 55 but were not suffering from dementia at the beginning of the study. They filled out questionnaires on what they ate each day.

The researchers worked out the percentage of processed and unprocessed foods the participants ate. They divided the participants into four groups and found that:

• Ultra-processed foods made up about a tenth of the daily diet of those in the lowest group—an average of 225 grams a day.

• Those in the highest group ate an average of 814 grams a day. Ultra-processed foods made up almost a third of their daily diet. A serving of fish sticks or pizza was equivalent to 150 grams. The major source of consumption for those in the groups with the highest levels of ultra-processed food was sodas. After that came sugary foods and ultra-processed dairy products.

• In the group that ate the *lowest* amount of processed food, 105 people developed dementia.

• In the group that ate the *highest* amount of processed food, 150 developed dementia.

The researchers concluded for every 10 percent increase in the amount of ultra-processed foods that they ate, the participants showed a 25 percent higher risk of developing dementia.

The study appears in the journal *Neurology*.

STEP SIX

Stay Away From Too Many Sugary Foods

This study underscores the theme of the importance of diet in the studies at which we have looked so far. This time, however, the substance to be avoided is fructose, a form of sugar.

It is a study with a difference. It comes up with a fascinating whole new way of looking at Alzheimer's and the role that sugary foods play in its development.

The research team at the University of Colorado Anschutz Medical Campus based their approach on how our ancient ancestors lived and how it has led to dementia today. They say that thousands of years ago our ancestors relied on fructose in the brain to help them forage for food. Fructose is a form of sugar that is found particularly in fruit and honey. Now, they say, that same instinct might be driving Alzheimer's disease.

For starters, the team approached the reasons for Alzheimer's as lying in what we eat.

"We make the case that Alzheimer's disease is driven by diet," says the study's lead author Dr Richard Johnson, who is a professor at the University of Colorado where the study was conducted. Johnson specializes in renal disease and hypertension.

The researchers go on to explain that they believe that Alzheimer's is a harmful adaptation of an evolutionary survival pathway that animals and our distant ancestors used when they faced a scarcity of food.

"A basic tenet of life is to assure enough food, water and oxygen for survival," the study says. "Much attention has focused on the acute survival responses to hypoxia and starvation. However, nature has developed a clever way to protect animals before the crisis usually occurs."

When early humans faced the possibility that they could starve, they developed a survival response that sent them foraging for food. Foraging is effective, however, only if the body's metabolism is inhibited. The reason is that, when they foraged, people needed focus, rapid assessment, impulsivity, exploratory behavior and risk taking.

Doing so was improved by blocking whatever got in the way, such as recent memories and attention to time. Fructose helped damp down those centers, allowing people to focus more on food gathering.

Indeed, the researchers found that the whole foraging response was boosted by fructose, whether it was eaten or produced in the body. So much so that fructose and its byproduct, intracellular uric acid, was critical to the survival of humans as well as animals.

The researchers found that fructose cuts the flow of blood to the cerebral cortex of the brain—that's the part involved in self-control—as well as the hippocampus and thalamus. At the same time, blood flow increased to the visual cortex that is linked with food reward.

Johnson explains that this whole process was reversible. In other words, once you stopped foraging for food you returned to normal and the blood flow returned to all the parts of your brain. But if it continues and becomes chronic, the result is brain decay and the loss of neurons. And that shows all the characteristics of Alzheimer's.

What Johnson calls the "survival switch" that was such a help in our ancestors when foraging for food has now become stuck in the "on" position. We tend to overeat high fat, sugary and salty food. And all that produces too much fructose. Too much fructose causes inflammation in the brain and eventually leads to Alzheimer's disease, the researchers found.

Here's an interesting twist: Johnson suspects that the tendency of some Alzheimer's patients to wander off might be a vestige of the ancient foraging response.

The message from the study is: Stop eating too many sugary foods and you will help to prevent developing dementia and Alzheimer's.

How The Study Was Conducted

The researchers tested their fructose theory on rats.

What they found was that when the rats were fed fructose for long enough, they developed tau and amyloid proteins in their brains—the same proteins seen in Alzheimer's disease.

"You can find high fructose levels in the brains of people with Alzheimer's as well," Johnson says.

The study is published in the *American Journal of Clinical Nutrition*.

STEP SEVEN

Two Australian studies link the quality of your sleep with your chances of suffering from dementia. Here's a look at both.

Ensure You Get Enough Deep Sleep

We all know sleep is essential for our general wellbeing and health. Now researchers in Australia have found that deep sleep plays a significant part in avoiding dementia.

They have found that even a one-percent reduction in deep sleep over a year can lead to a 27 percent increase in the risk of dementia of those who are older than 60.

So what is deep sleep? Also called "slow-wave sleep" it is the third stage of non-REM sleep and is essential if we want to wake up feeling refreshed and rested.

Deep sleep is characterized by lower brain wave activity, slower breathing and a slower heart rate. It usually lasts around an hour or an hour-and-a-half and takes place early in the night.

"Slow-wave sleep, or deep sleep, supports the aging brain in many ways, and we know that sleep augments the clearance of metabolic waste from the brain, including facilitating the clearance of proteins that aggregate in Alzheimer's disease," says Associate Professor Matthew Pase of the Monash School of Psychological Sciences and the Turner Institute for Brain and Mental Health in Melbourne, Australia.

"However, to date we have been unsure of the role of slow-wave sleep in the development of dementia. Our findings suggest that slow wave sleep loss may be a modifiable dementia risk factor."

The study found that the amount of deep sleep we have lessens as we age. The researchers fail to explain in the study how you are supposed to ensure that you obtain sufficient deep sleep when you get older.

Pase did say, however, that a genetic risk factor for Alzheimer's disease, but not brain volume, was associated with accelerated declines in slow-wave sleep.

How The Study Was Conducted

The study looked at 346 participants aged more than 60 in the Framingham Heart Study who completed two overnight sleep studies from 1995 to 1998 and 2001 to 2003, with an average of five years between the two studies.

The participants were carefully followed for dementia from the time of the second sleep study through to 2018. The researchers found that, on average, the amount of deep sleep dropped between the two studies, indicating that the amount of deep sleep decreased as the participants grew older.

During the 17 years of follow-up 52 cases of dementia took place.

Even adjusting for age, sex, cohort, genetic factors, smoking status, use of sleep medication, use of antidepressants and anxiety drug use, each percentage decrease in deep sleep was associated with a 27 percent increase in the risk of dementia each year, the study found.

The study is published in *JAMA Neurology.*

Keep To Regular Sleep Patterns

The other sleep study found that people who have a highly irregular sleep pattern might have as much as a 53 percent higher risk of dementia than those who have more regular sleep patterns.

The researchers emphasize that the study does not prove sleep irregularity causes dementia, but it shows a link between the two.

Regular sleep is consistently going to sleep and waking at the same times each day.

"Sleep health recommendations often focus on getting the recommended amount of sleep—which is seven to nine hours a night—but there is less emphasis on maintaining regular sleep schedules," says Monash University's Dr. Matthew Pase, who also wrote this study as well as the previously cited one on deep sleep.

 "Our findings suggest the regularity of a person's sleep is an important factor when considering a person's risk of dementia."

He suggests that, based on the research team's findings, people with irregular sleep patterns need only to improve their sleep regularity to average levels, compared with extremely high levels, to prevent dementia.

How The Study Was Conducted

This study involved 88,094 people aged an average 62 in the United Kingdom. They were followed for an average seven years.

Those who took part wore a wrist device for seven day that measured their sleep cycle. Researchers then calculated the regularity of their sleep. A person who sleeps and wakes at the same times every day would have a sleep regularity index of 100. A person who sleeps and wakes at different times every day would have a score of zero.

The researchers found that 480 participants developed dementia. They compared those with an average sleep regularity index with those who failed to do so. They found the risk of dementia was highest for people who had the most irregular sleep.

People in the lowest fifth percentile had he most irregular sleep with an average score of 41. Those in the highest 95th percentile had the most regular sleep with a score of 71. Those between the two groups scored an average 60.

After adjusting for age, sex and genetic risk of Alzheimer's disease, researchers found that those with the most irregular sleep were 53 percent more likely to develop dementia than those in the middle group.

The study is published in *Neurology,* the American Journal of Neurology.

STEP EIGHT

Be Active

A secret to lowering your chances of dementia when you are older is to be active—particularly in your community—when you are younger. The more active you are, the more likely you are to keep your brain active. That is the finding in a study at Brighton and Sussex Medical School in England.

Your activity might be taking part in artistic activities, playing sport, joining a local club, volunteering for a community project or joining a religious group. Even having a stimulating job, going to college, reading, gardening, completing puzzles, or playing board games can play a role. Listening to the radio and visiting museums also help.

Going to college does not mean only heading to school in your early years. Continuing to learn over a lifetime provides a buffer against conditions such as Alzheimer's—even for those who perform poorly at school. Such activity assists your brain in storing "healthy neurons," the study finds.

"These results are exciting because they indicate cognitive ability is subject to factors throughout our lifetimes and taking part in an intellectually, socially and physically active lifestyle might help to ward off cognitive decline and dementia," says Dr. Dorina Cadar of the Brighton and Sussex Medical School.

"It's heartening to find that building up one's cognitive reserve may offset the negative influence of low childhood cognition for people who might not have benefited from an enriching childhood and offer stronger mental resilience until later."

How The Study Was Conducted

A total of 1,184 people who were born in 1946 in the United Kingdom were involved in the study.

They took cognitive tests when they were eight years old and again when they were 69. An index combined their educational level at age 26, participation in enriching leisure activities at 69 and occupations up to age 53. Their reading ability at age 53 was also tested as a measure of overall lifelong learning separate from education and occupation.

The participants took a brain test at age 69. It has a maximum score of 100. The average for the group was 92. The lowest score was 53 and the highest 100. The researchers found that higher childhood cognitive skills, a higher cognitive reserve index and a higher reading ability were all linked to higher scores on the test.

Those people with a bachelor's degree or higher scored 1.22 points more on average than those with no formal education. People who took part in six or more leisure activities—such as clubs, volunteer work, adult education classes, social activities and gardening— scored 1.53 points more on average than people who engaged in up to four leisure activities. Those with a professional or intermediate level job scored 1.5 points more than those with partly skilled or unskilled occupations.

The study appears in the journal *Neurology*.

STEP NINE

Adopt A Positive Outlook On Life
And Be Socially Interactive

A related study also found that your lifestyle has a lot to do in determining whether you will develop dementia when you are older.

Those people who are more organized, have a positive outlook on life, work hard and display a high degree of self-discipline are less likely to suffer from the disease, the study at the University of Victoria in British Columbia, Canada found.

Their research was part of an international study conducted by researchers at the University of Victoria as well as Northwestern University in Evanston, Illinois; Rush University Medical Center, Chicago; and the University of Edinburgh in Scotland.

The study found that drifting toward dementia or Alzheimer's disease can be turned around if you become less stressed and more socially active when you are older. Positive personality characteristics might protect a person even after they start to develop dementia, the scientists found.

Personality characteristics reflect patterns of thinking and behavior that are long-lasting, according to Dr. Tomiko Yoneda of the University of Victoria who helped conduct the study.

The cumulative impact of these characteristics affect the way in which we engage in healthy or unhealthy activities over our lifetimes.

These experiences make you more or less susceptible to developing certain diseases or disorders, such as mild brain impairment, Yoneda says. They also mean that some people can resist changes in the brain that are connected with aging whereas other people are less able to do so.

The study shows that being socially interactive can help to improve your brain health even later in life, notes Yoneda.

How The Study Was Conducted

A total of 1,954 people took part in the study of older people who live in the greater Chicago metropolitan area and northeastern Illinois. None of the participants was formally diagnosed with dementia when the study began in 1977. They were chosen from retirement communities, church groups and senior housing facilities.

In the study the researchers rated the participants on personality characteristics. They then tested those characteristics against the development of brain impairment when they became older.

The researchers divided the participants into three main groups.

1. **Those who scored high on conscientiousness.**

These were people who view life in a positive light. They are hard-working and diligent. They tend to be responsible, organized and work toward reaching goals in life.

2. **Those who scored high on neuroticism.**

These people have lower emotional stability. They tend toward mood swings, anxiety, self-doubt, depression and negative feelings.

3. **Those who scored high on being extroverts.**

These people gain energy from being with others. They direct their energy toward the outside world, tending to be enthusiastic, gregarious, talkative and assertive.

The research team found that the group that scored high on conscientiousness and those who scored low on neuroticism were less likely to suffer mild brain impairment when they became older.

At the opposite end of the spectrum, those who scored low on conscientiousness and high on neuroticism were more likely to suffer brain impairment later in life. No link was found between those who scored high on extroversion and brain impairment.

Those who scored high on extroversion—as well as those who scored high on consciousness and low on neuroticism—tended to maintain normal brain functioning longer than the others.

The study is in the *Journal of Personality and Social Psychology*.

STEP 10

Act Younger Than You Are

This study takes the lifestyle approach in the previous study a little further. It suggests that we should be measured by our biological age rather than our chronological age. If we are, those who are biologically younger are less likely to develop dementia.

We all know people who look and act a lot older—and those who look and act a lot younger—than they really are.

The study at the Karolinska Institutet in Stockholm, Sweden found that a higher biological age (when you appear older than you really are) is linked to a significantly higher risk of dementia.

"If a person's biological age is five years higher than their actual age, the person has a 40 percent higher risk of developing vascular dementia or suffering a stroke," says Jonathan Mak, a doctoral student at the Department of Medical Epidemiology and Biostatistics at the institution.

How The Study Was Conducted

The researchers ran their tests on 325,000 people. They were aged between 40 and 70 when the study began.

They calculated their biological ages using 18 biomarkers, including blood sugar, blood pressure, blood lipids, lung function and weight (bodily mass index or BMI).

They watched the people in the study for nine years and assessed the risk of developing dementia and other neurodegenerative diseases over a period of nine years.

They concluded that, when compared with actual chronological age, a higher biological age (when you appear older than you real age) was linked with a significantly increased risk of dementia.

The study is published in *BMJ Journals*.

STEP 11

Exercise Regularly

Exercise helps to prevent dementia, according to a study by researchers at Inserm Research Center in Caen, France.

Their studies show that exercise protects brain volume. It also lowers a person's weight and keeps insulin levels low, both of which can help to promote brain health.

"These results might help us to understand how physical activity affects brain health, which might guide us in developing strategies to prevent or delay age-related decline in memory and thinking skills, says Dr. Géraldine Poisnel who works at the research center. "Older adults who are physically active gain cardiovascular benefits, which might result in greater structural brain integrity."

Previous studies also have shown that exercise helps protect your brain cells.

The investigators say more research is needed to understand the mechanisms behind these regulations.

"Maintaining a lower BMI (bodily mass index) through physical activity could help prevent disturbed insulin metabolism that is often seen in aging, thus promoting brain health," Poisnel says.

How The Study Was Conducted

A total of 134 individuals, averaging age 69, who did not have memory problems were included in the study.

They completed questionnaires about their physical activity for the previous year. They also underwent brain scans that measured their glucose metabolism and brain volume.

The researchers also gathered information about their blood pressure, weight (BMI or bodily mass index), insulin levels, and other factors.

The investigators found that those people in the study with the most physical activity had higher total volumes of gray matter in their brain than those with the least amount of physical activity.

When they examined areas of the brain that were affected by Alzheimer's disease, they found similar results.

The study did not prove that exercise protects brain volume, but investigators say they found a link between the two.

The study is published in *Science Daily.*

Exercise Improves Brain Health

Another new study supports the finding that regular exercise lowers the risk of dementia.

Research by a team of clinical researchers from Pacific Neuroscience Institute's Brain Health Center in Santa Monica finds that being physically active relates to improved brain health.

"Our research supports earlier studies that show being physically active is good for your brain," says Dr. Cyrus A. Raji, the lead researcher. "Exercise not only lowers the risk of dementia but also helps in maintaining brain size, which is crucial as we age."

Fewer Than 4,000 Steps

A fascinating finding in this study is that even moderate levels of activity, such as taking fewer than 4,000 steps a day, can have a modest effect on brain health, says Dr. David Merrill, co-author of the study and director of the institute. This is far less than the regularly suggested 10,000 steps, he says, making it a more achievable goal for many people.

"Our research links regular physical activity to larger brain volumes, suggesting neuro-protective benefits," explains study co-author Dr Somayeh Meysami, assistant professor of neurosciences at Saint John's Cancer Institute and the Pacific Brain Health Center. "This large sample study furthers our understanding of lifestyle factors in brain health and dementia prevention.

"This study...when added to other studies on the role of diet, stress reduction, and social connection offers the proven benefits of drug-free modifiable factors in substantially reducing Alzheimer's disease," says George Perry, editor-in-chief of the *Journal of Alzheimer's Disease.*

The research highlights an easy way to keep our brain healthy: stay active, the research team says. Whether it is a daily walk or a favorite sport, regular physical activity can have lasting benefits for our brain health.

How The Study Was Conducted

The researchers looked at MRI brain scans from 10,125 people at Prenuvo imaging centers.

It found those who regularly engaged in physical activities, such as walking, running or sports, had larger brain volumes in key areas. This includes the gray matter, which helps with processing information, and the white matter, which connects different brain regions, as well as the hippocampus, which is important for memory.

The study appears in the *Journal of Alzheimer's disease.*

STEP 12

Maintain Healthy Habits

Conducted at the University of Mississippi Medical Center in Jackson, this study suggests that seven healthy habits and lifestyle factors play a role in lowering the risk of dementia in people generally —and even those with the highest genetic risk.

The seven healthy habits—known as the American Heart Association's Life's Simple 7—are:

1. Stop Smoking

2. Eat Better

3. Get Active

4. Lose Weight

5. Manage Blood Pressure

6. Control Cholesterol

7. Reduce Blood Sugar

"These healthy habits in Life's Simple 7 have been linked (in earlier studies) to a lower risk of dementia overall, but it was uncertain whether the same applies to people with a high genetic risk," says Dr. Adrienne Tin of the University of Mississippi Medical Center in Jackson, the author of the study.

"The good news is that even for people who are at the highest genetic risk, living by this same healthier lifestyle are likely to have a lower risk of dementia."

You can learn more about Life's Simple 7 and dementia at BrainandLife.org, home of the American Academy of Neurology's free patient and caregiver magazine which focuses on the intersection of neurologic disease and brain health.

How The Study Was Conducted

The study looked at 8,823 people of European ancestry and 2,738 people of African ancestry. They had an average age of 54 at the start of the study. They were followed for 30 years.

Researchers calculated genetic risk scores at the beginning of the study using genome-wide statistics of Alzheimer's disease.

Those with European ancestry were divided into five groups and those with African ancestry into three groups, based on genetic risk scores.

By the end of the study 1,603 people with European ancestry and 631 people with African ancestry developed dementia.

For those with European ancestry the researchers found that people with the highest scores in the lifestyle factors had a lower risk of dementia across all five genetic risk groups. For every one-point increase in the lifestyle factor score there was a 9 percent lower risk of developing dementia.

Among those with European ancestry, the intermediate and high categories were linked with a 30 percent and 43 percent lower risk for dementia than those in the low category of the lifestyle factor score.

Among those with African ancestry, the intermediate and high categories were linked to a 6 percent and 17 percent lower risk for dementia.

Those in whom the two proteins were found were considered to be at a 20 to 40 percent higher risk of developing dementia when they were followed up a few years later, compared with those participants who had no such changes.

The study appears in the journal *Neurobiology.*

Wrapping It Up

A recently published wide-ranging study at the University of Exeter in England and Maastricht University in the Netherlands wraps up much of what has been found in other studies.

The research followed more than 350,000 participants younger than 65 across the United Kingdom from the UK Biobank.

The team took a close look at a wide range of risk factors ranging from genetic predispositions to lifestyle and environmental influences.

The study showed that lower formal education, lower socioeconomic status, genetic variation, lifestyle factors such as alcohol use disorder and social isolation, and health issues including vitamin D deficiency, depression, stroke, hearing impairment and heart disease significantly elevate risk of what the researchers call "young-onset dementia."

The study is the largest and most robust of its kind ever conducted, says Professor David Llewellyn of the University of Exeter. "It reveals that we may be able to take action to reduce risk of this debilitating condition through targeting a range of different factors."

Such factors are outlined in this report.

The study is published in *JAMA Neurology*.

DEMENTIA TESTS

Those, then, are the 12 steps. Each lowers your risk of developing dementia to a certain degree. If you follow them all, therefore, your chances of evading dementia must be considered to be reasonably high.

Clearly, too, if you can find out that you are susceptible to dementia as long as 20 years in advance, you would want to be absolutely sure to take these steps.

To close, therefore, we take a look at what is happening in the field of advance tests.

Early Detection

Alzheimer's disease can be detected up to 20 years before you are aware of any symptoms, such as memory loss, according to a large international study led by scientists at Sweden's Lund University.

Changes in your brain take place before symptoms appear, the scientists say. They involve the two proteins—beta-amyloid, which lays down plaque in the brain, and tau, which grows over time inside brain cells.

It is only when the tau begins to spread that nerve cells die, explains Dr. Oskar Hansson, a senior neurology physician at Skåne Hospital. The person then starts to experience the first symptoms, such as loss of memory. The slow build-up over time is a reason that it is so difficult to diagnose Alzheimer's disease in its early stages.

Such findings also point the way to a person being able to take steps to prevent the disease before it takes hold.

Hansson led a large international research study with 1,325 participants from Sweden, the United States , the Netherlands, and Australia.

The participants had no brain impairment at the start of the study. The researchers used pet scans to see the presence of tau and amyloid in the participants' brains.

Those in whom the two proteins were found were considered to be at a 20 to 40 percent higher risk of developing dementia when they were followed up a few years later, compared with those participants who had no such changes.

"When both beta-amyloid and tau are present in the brain, it can no longer be considered a risk factor, but rather a diagnosis," says Risk Ossenkoppele, who is a senior researcher at Lund University and Amsterdam University Medical Center.

"A pathologist who examines samples from a brain like this would immediately diagnose the patient with Alzheimer's."

He adds that the results of the study can be compared with prostate cancer. If a doctor performs a biopsy and finds cancer cells the diagnosis will be cancer, even if the person in question has not yet developed any symptoms. Based on this, the study at Lund University is particularly interesting, he says.

Such findings also point the way to a person being able to take steps, such as physical activity and good nutrition, to prevent the disease before it takes hold, Hansson says.

The study appears in the journal *Nature Medicine*.

Screening Test

Scientists at the Karolinska Institutet in Stockholm Sweden found that a type of sugar molecule in your blood is linked with the level of tau, a protein that plays a critical role in the development of severe dementia.

The study paves the way for a simple screening procedure that will be able to predict the onset of dementia and Alzheimer's as long as 10 years in advance using a blood test and a simple memory test.

The researchers in this study say that in Alzheimer's disease the neurons of the brain die. The reason for this is believed to be the result of the abnormal accumulation of two proteins, amyloid beta and tau.

Trials have found that treatment should start early in the process, before too many neurons have died, to reverse the process before it is too late.

The researchers found that the level of a certain glycan structure in a person's blood denotes the presence of what is called bisected N-acetylglucosamine, which can be used to predict the risk of developing Alzheimer's disease.

Previous tests to determine the presence of this substance were conducted on fluid in the brain which is more difficult and expensive to test. Markers in blood are preferable.

"We're collaborating with researchers in primary care in Sweden to evaluate different biomarkers for dementia at primary health care centres," says Dr. Schedin Weiss, a docent at NVS, Karolinksa Institut. "We hope that glycans in the blood will prove to be a valuable complement to current methods of screening people for Alzheimer's disease that will enable the disease to be detected early."

The study is published in *Alzheimer's & Dementia*, the journal of the Alzheimer's Association.

Saliva Test

Scientists at the University of Alberta in Canada say they are working on developing a saliva test for Alzheimer's disease. Such a test would prove useful because it is easy and non-invasive, they say. It also has the potential to detect neurodegenerative diseases at an early stage, allowing for steps to be taken early to lower the risk for the disease.

"So far, no disease-altering interventions for Alzheimer's disease have been successful, explains Dr. Roger Dixon, a professor in the Department of Psychology at the university. "For this reason, researchers are aiming to discover the earliest signals of the disease so that prevention protocols can be implemented."

In other words, should the saliva test successfully identify people who are liable to contract Alzheimer's disease later in life, they will be able to take steps such as those outlined in this report to ward off the disease or at least delay its occurrence.

The research is published in the *Journal of Alzheimer's Disease* as well as in *Frontiers in Aging Neuroscience*.

A Final Note

Thank you for reading this publication. We hope it helps you determine how you can avoid developing dementia—or at least sharply lower your risks of doing so—by acting early in your life or even when you are older.

Following these steps also is likely to lead to generally healthier living and contribute toward reducing your chances of suffering a stroke or a heart attack as well.

We would like to thank those scientists, too, who spent a considerable amount of time, money and effort in conducting the studies that led to these findings.

Next Steps

We have put together a list of books, recipes and other helpful content that you might wish to read as well as links to the studies in medical journals cited in this report.

They can be found at https://www.dotcash.com/dementia